20th Century Inventions

MEDICAL ADVANCES

Steve Parker

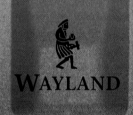

WAYLAND

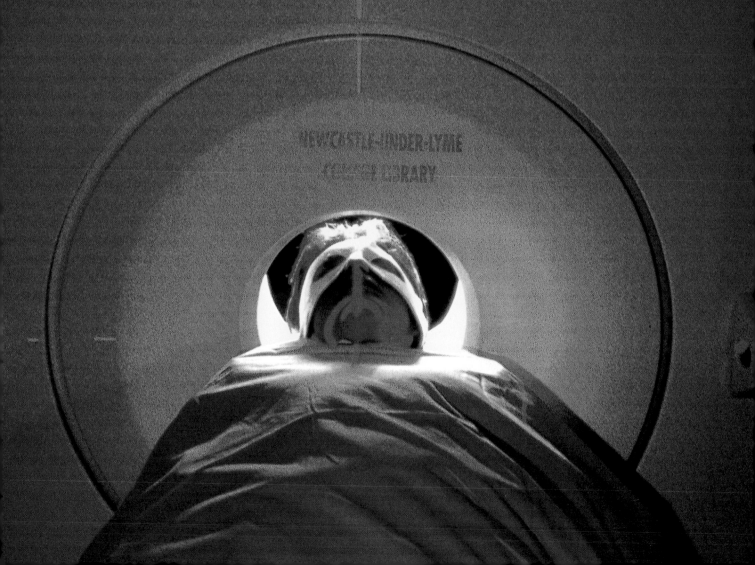

20th Century Inventions

AIRCRAFT

CARS

COMPUTERS

THE INTERNET

LASERS

NUCLEAR POWER

ROCKETS AND SPACECRAFT

SATELLITES

TELECOMMUNICATIONS

Front cover and title page: A patient undergoing a PET brain scan (see page 19)
Back cover: MRI scan of a brain (see page 18)
Series editor: Philippa Smith
Book editor: Jannet King
Series designer: Tim Mayer
Book designer: Malcolm Walker of Kudos Design
Cover designer: Dennis Day

First published in 1997 by Wayland Publishers Limited,
61 Western Road, Hove, East Sussex BN3 1JD, England

© Copyright 1997 Wayland Publishers Limited

Find Wayland on the internet at http://www.wayland.co.uk

British Library Cataloguing in Publication Data
Parker, Steve, 1952–
    Medical Advances. – (Twentieth century inventions)
    1. Medical technology – Juvenile literature 2.Medical technology – History – 20th
century – Juvenile literature
    I. Title
    610.2'8

ISBN 0 7502 2096 1

Typeset by Malcolm Walker
Printed and bound in Italy by G. Canale & C.S.p.A., Turin

Picture acknowledgements
Bubbles 43 (bottom)/James Lamb; Hulton Getty Picture Library:
6 (top), 8, 9 (top) & (bottom), 44 (top), (bottom); Image Select:
7, 12 (bottom)/Jean Mohr; Impact: 5 (top)/Caroline Penn,
41/Mike McQueen; Science Photo Library: front cover & title
page/Hank Morgan, back cover & contents page/Scott
Camazine, 4/Jim Olive, Peter Arnold Inc, 5 (bottom)/Volger
Steger, Peter Arnold Inc, 6 (bottom)/Mark de Fraeye/World View,
10 (top)/Saturn Stills & bottom/ Blair Seitz, 11/Saturn Stills, 12
(top)/CC Studio, 13/Simon Fraser, 14/Eye of Science, 15
(top)/Philippe Plailly & bottom/Robert Longuehaye, NIBSC,
16/Philippe Plailly, 18/Simon Fraser,19 (top)/Will & Deni
McIntyre & (bottom)/Mehau Kulyk, 20/CC Studio, 21 (top)/Jerry
Mason & (bottom)/Robert Holmgren, Peter Arnold Inc, 22/D Vo
Trung/Eurelios, 23/Alexander Tsiaras, 24, 25/J C Revy, 27/Adam
Hart-Davis, 29/John Greim, 30 (top)/Custom Medical Stock
Photo & (bottom)/Will & Deni McIntyre, 31/Hank Morgan,
32/Alexander Tsiaras, 33/, 34 (top)/Mehau Kulyk &
(bottom)/Hank Morgan, 35/Princess Margaret Rose Hostpial,
36/Claude Charlier, 37/Geoff Tompkinson, 38/Chris Priest &
Mark Clarke, 39/Russell D Curtis, 40/Philippe Plailly,
42/Philippe Plailly, 43 (top)/James King-Holmes & , 45/Will &
Deni McIntyre; Shout 26, 28; Artwork by Tim Benké, Top Draw
(Tableaux) 13, 17, 18, 23

20th Century Inventions
CONTENTS

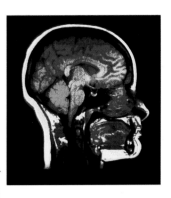

INTRODUCTION

When were you last ill? In the world's richer countries, most people are well for most of the time. Although we have minor illnesses, such as colds and sore throats, we soon recover from them. Some people have more serious, longer-term conditions, such as asthma, diabetes and kidney disease. These can often be kept under control with modern drugs, medical machines and other advanced treatments. A few people, though, suffer very serious health conditions, such as certain forms of cancer. Their outlook is less certain.

So what is medicine? It involves preventing diseases, relieving pain and suffering, treating sickness, healing illness and disease, and restoring health. Just as there is a huge range of illness and disease, there is also a huge range of medical methods and treatments. These have changed vastly through history, and today they still vary enormously around the world.

A person's life is priceless. But there are limits on the price we can afford for medical care. The helicopter air-ambulance costs thousands of pounds per life-saving trip. Yet this money could save dozens of lives if spent in other ways.

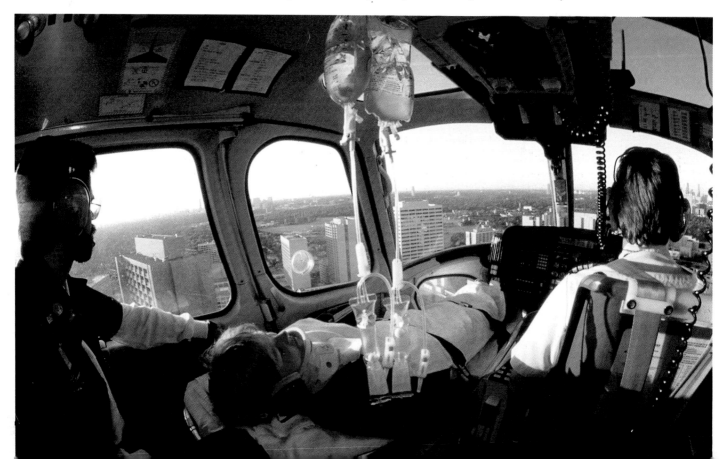

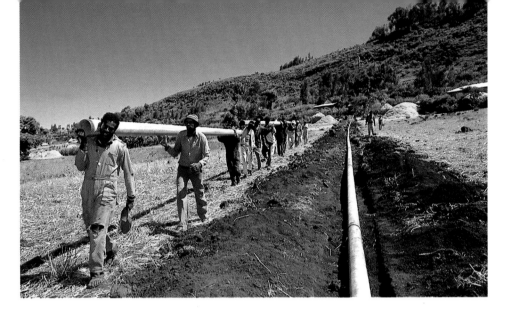

Villagers in Ethiopia lay a pipeline for clean water. This is one of the most basic needs for health, and also an extremely cost-effective way of fighting illness. Many dangerous diseases, such as typhoid and cholera, are spread by germs in contaminated water.

Health problems in poorer countries

In many countries in the world the medical care that we take for granted is just not available. Although traditional medicine can be effective in treating certain conditions, millions of people in poorer countries still suffer and die from a whole range of illnesses that could be easily treated and cured if there was money to pay for medical care.

Infections caused by germs are particularly common in poorer countries. They spread rapidly where there are unhygienic living conditions, dirty water, parasites and pests, lack of understanding about health and illness and little nourishing food.

The 20th century

In terms of easing suffering, and saving lives, by far the biggest medical changes have come about in the 20th century. They are based on scientific research and scientific methods developed in the richer, industrialized countries. They involve improved living conditions, better understanding of disease, more preventative medicine, immunizations, new drugs, the latest surgical methods, and even the occasional chance discovery – as described in this book.

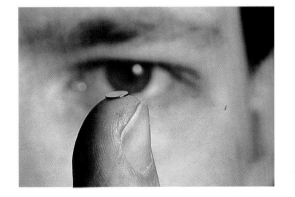

Medicine as part of science

Medicine is not separate from other branches of science. Advances in many scientific areas help medicine, and the reverse. For example, modern body scanners would not be possible without powerful computers. Spare parts, such as artificial joints, rely on the skills of materials scientists and hi-tech bio-engineering. While genetic experts exchange information across many scientific areas, from medicine to wildlife conservation.

At the forefront of electronic medicine is the retinal implant. It changes light energy into electrical signals, similar to the body's nerve impulses. Put into the eye, it could help blind people to see.

Ancient and medieval medicine

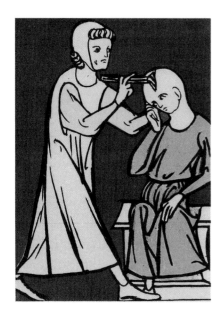

Above **The smooth-shafted, metal-tipped trepanning drill, like a thick arrow, was an early piece of medical technology. Trepanning was probably intended to release 'evil spirits' from the head, which people believed caused odd behaviour or severe headaches that we now call migraine.**

Medicine has existed since the Stone Age. Human skulls, more than 10,000 years old, have been found with holes chipped or drilled into them – a practice called trepanning. The bones show signs that they healed, so the patients obviously lived through the procedure!

Ancient medicine

By the time of Ancient Mesopotamia, Egypt, India and China (some 3,000 to 5,000 years ago), there were people who specialized in medicine – physicians. Some of the medicines prescribed then are still being used now. Chinese herbal medicine and the technique of acupuncture (sticking needles into the skin) has a history stretching back several thousands of years and both are still used to great effect nowadays. Indeed, they are sometimes used in the West in addition to conventional western medicine. Such techniques are known here as complementary medicine.

Right **Traditional remedies are still prepared in their thousands and used by millions of people, especially in South and East Asia, and South America. This selection from Taiwan includes some cast snakes' skins.**

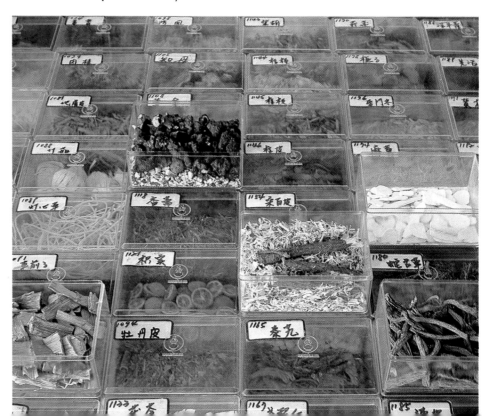

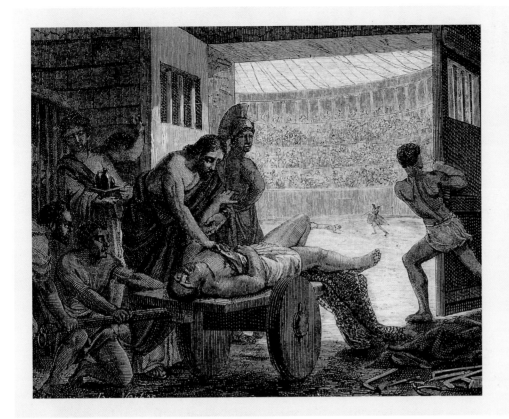

Ancient Rome's foremost physician was Claudius Galen (AD **130–200**). His many books explained how the body works and how to treat illnesses. Custom did not allow people to be cut open deliberately, either for research or treatment, but Galen was physician to the gladiators who fought terrible battles in the Colosseum, so he saw plenty of human innards.

The birth of modern medicine

One of the best-known early physicians was Hippocrates (460–377 BC) of Ancient Greece. He brought some common sense to medicine, teaching that the body often has the power to heal itself. Ill people should rest and eat good food, and the physician should look for the cause of disease, treat it, but otherwise interfere as little as possible. Doctors have been guided by his thinking ever since.

Types of treatments

These early physicans used three types of treatment on their patients, sometimes all at the same time. One kind of treatment involved giving the patient chemical substances from nature, especially herbs and plant extracts, rare minerals from the rocks, and even animal products such as ox urine and lizard droppings. These were the first drugs. Another kind was physical treatment, including cutting bits out of, or off, the body with a sharp blade – the first surgery. The third type of treatment involved magical and religious prayers and chants, to ask for the help of the gods and spirits.

The medical revolution

Until the fifteenth century in Europe, physicians treated patients according to age-old traditions, mixing medicine with magic and religion. But in the sixteenth century Andreas Vesalius, in Padua, Italy, went against custom and dissected dead bodies in order to study organs and tissues. His work *On the Structure of the Human Body*, first published in 1543, is the basis of modern medical anatomy.

A scientific approach

In the early seventeenth century people such as Galileo Galilei argued that scientists should be free to propose ideas and theories, carry out tests and experiments, measure and analyse the results, and make discoveries and inventions. This scientific method for advancing knowledge and understanding was soon being applied to medicine.

From about 1600 onwards microscopes were used to reveal the tiny world of cells and germs. In 1628 the experiments of the English physician William Harvey showed that an age-old belief was mistaken. Blood was not continually made and used up; it flowed round and round the body, pumped by the heart.

A lucky discovery

One of the greatest advances in medicine was Alexander Fleming's 1928 discovery of the first antibiotic – a drug that kills bacteria germs. Fleming was experimenting with bacteria growing in dishes. He went on holiday, leaving one dish uncovered. On return, he noticed a fungus or mould had settled on the dish and killed the bacteria. The fungus was *Penicillium* and the drug made from it was named penicillin. Antibiotics have since saved millions of lives.

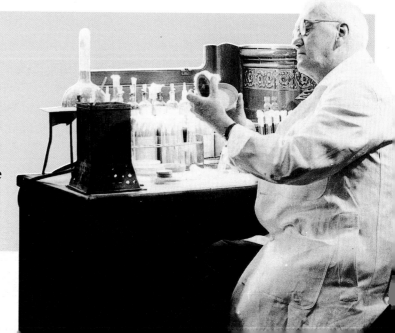

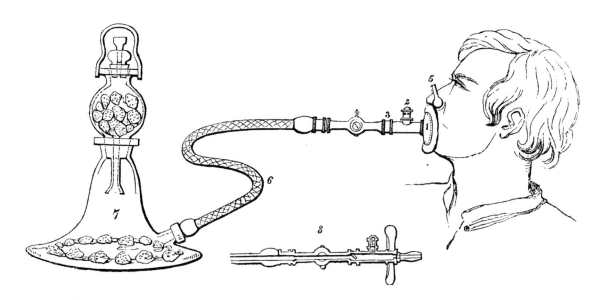

Above **In this early anaesthetic apparatus, from about 1847, the patient lost consciousness while breathing ether gas, from the ether-soaked sponges in the jar. Within a few years, chloroform replaced ether.**

Better surgery

In 1846 American doctor–dentist William Morton was the first to use anaesthesia for an operation, to 'send the patient to sleep'. In the 1860s English surgeon Joseph Lister began the use of germ-killing antiseptics during operations. A patient's chances of surviving surgery improved from 1-in-2 to 19-in-20.

Seeing into the body

Progress in other areas of science helped medicine. In 1895 German physics professor Wilhem Röntgen discovered new invisible rays. They passed through soft substances like flesh, but not through hard, dense substances such as bones. He called them X-rays – 'X' for 'unknown'. Within weeks they were being used to detect broken bones and other internal problems. This was the beginning of medical imaging.

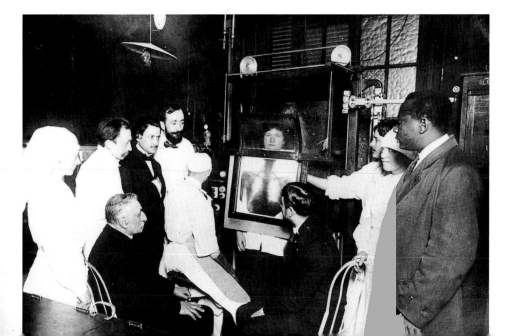

Left **This X-ray apparatus, from about 1900, shows the woman's chest bones 'live on screen'. People were not aware of X-rays' harmful effects. In today's equipment, the rays are more controlled and less powerful, and there are precautions and protective clothing for patients and operators.**

PREVENTING ILLNESS

Many older designs of medical equipment are being replaced by smaller, microchip-controlled versions. The electronic blood pressure monitor measures blood pressure automatically and continuously. It gives a digital read-out and even a paper print-out.

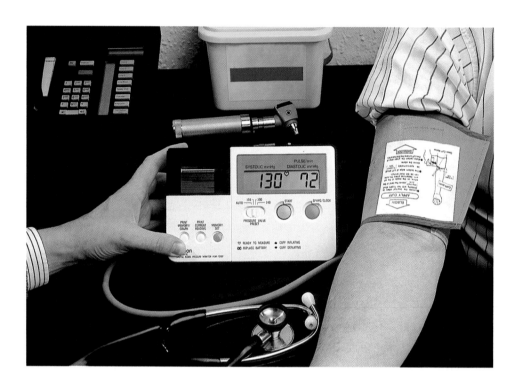

Hippocrates of Ancient Greece taught that preventing illness, or detecting it early on, is better than trying to treat it late. Doctors follow this idea today, using a wide variety of sophisticated machines and methods. However, some older inventions for checking health are still most useful. The clinical thermometer, which measures body temperature, dates back to the 1880s, as does the manual sphygmomanometer, for measuring blood pressure.

ECG machine

A check-up on an ECG (electro-cardiograph) machine can warn of heart problems (see also page 21). Tiny electrical signals, passing out from the pumping heart, are detected on the skin and displayed as a wavy line. In the 1900s early ECG machines filled whole rooms. Today's portable ECG is as small as a laptop computer.

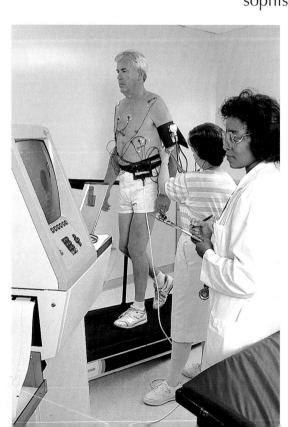

An exercise ECG monitors the electrical signals of the heart, which pumps harder and faster as the person walks or runs on a treadmill.

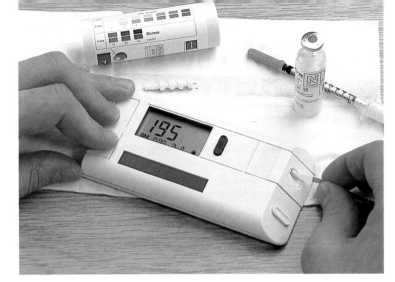

Taking samples

Besides physical and electrical tests, there are hundreds of different kinds of chemical tests. These are done on various samples from the body: strands of hair, skin scrapings, nasal mucus, phlegm, sputum, urine, faeces, and blood removed with a needle and syringe. They also include cervical mucus from the neck of the womb (taken during a cervical smear test), synovial fluid from a joint, even cerebrospinal fluid from inside the brain. Biopsy samples of flesh and tissues can also be taken from muscle, liver, bone marrow and intestinal lining. The samples are usually sent to the local medical laboratory for analysis (see page 24).

Raised blood glucose, or sugar, may signal the condition called diabetes. Diabetic people can now monitor their condition themselves at home, using a small hand-held blood glucose meter. It helps them to fine-tune their treatment – a controlled diet, tablets, insulin injections, or possibly a combination of all three.

Information in blood

Blood can be tested for a wide range of signs of ill-health, including raised cholesterol. This fatty substance is vital for health but, if too plentiful, can clog blood vessels and maybe lead to a heart attack. People identified as at risk can take preventative measures, such as changing their eating habits.

Screening

Screening detects conditions that might not yet show any obvious signs. Testing everyone for everything would be impossible, so the range of conditions tested is narrowed down, for example, to conditions that:
• can be treated or cured (otherwise there's little point in detection)
• can be detected early, in a relatively simple way
• tend to occur in certain target groups of people.
The cervical smear test, in which cells taken from the neck of the womb are analysed, is carried out every few years on women over a certain age. It detects early changes which could lead to cancer. Mammography, a specialized type of X-ray, detects tumours (growths) in the breast.

Protecting against disease

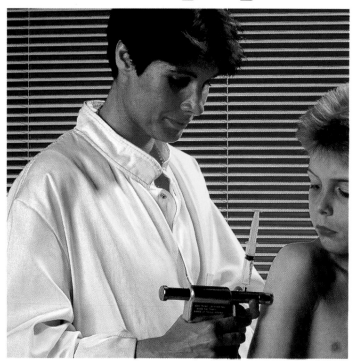

In the 1790s English physician Edward Jenner showed that deliberately giving someone the disease cowpox made them resistant or immune to the more serious version of the disease, smallpox. Much scientific work since has led to immunization being increasingly safe and effective against certain diseases. It has saved untold lives and ranks as one of the greatest medical advances of all time.

The vaccine gun automatically injects the correct amount of vaccine, to give protection against certain infectious diseases.

Basics of immunity

If the body catches certain germs, such as measles, its immune system fights them. Microscopic white cells in the blood attack them directly, or make antibodies that destroy them. This causes illness. Hopefully, the body wins the battle and 'remembers' that type of germ in the future. If it invades again, the system's white cells destroy it before it causes illness. We call this being protected against, or immune to, the illness.

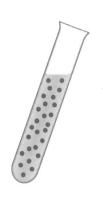

A vaccine can be made by injecting animals with an infection and purifying their blood, or from genetically engineered bacteria.

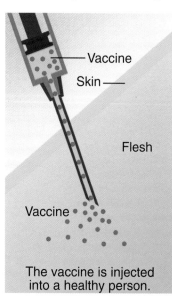

Vaccine
Skin
Flesh
Vaccine

The vaccine is injected into a healthy person.

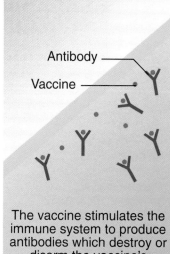

Antibody
Vaccine

The vaccine stimulates the immune system to produce antibodies which destroy or disarm the vaccine's disabled germs.

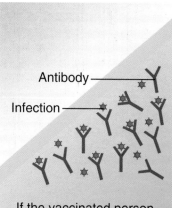

Antibody
Infection

If the vaccinated person is in contact with the infection, they already have the antibodies that recognize, and can fight against, the real germs!

Common immunizations

The exact types and timing of immunization vary, depending on diseases in an area, and vaccines and staff available. In Western countries they may include:

- **DTP** – against diphtheria, tetanus and pertussis (whooping cough), as a combined injection
- **MMR** – against measles, mumps and rubella (german measles), as a combined injection
- **Polio** – against polio, as a drop
- **BCG** – against tuberculosis, TB, as an injection
- **Tetanus** – against tetanus or 'lockjaw', by injection, boosted every 5–10 years

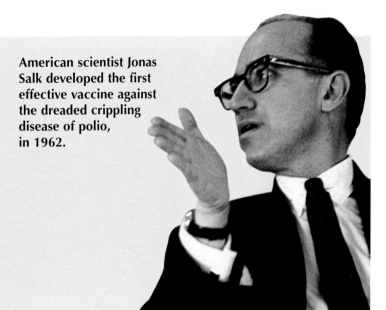

American scientist Jonas Salk developed the first effective vaccine against the dreaded crippling disease of polio, in 1962.

Immunization

Vaccines contain specially killed or weakened forms of germs. Put into the body, in vaccination, they cause not illness, but immunity. Immunization is usually carried out early in life, before real germs invade. It is effective only against certain germs, however. Also, if a person has already suffered certain diseases, or if certain conditions run in the family, a particular immunization may be advised against, because it could do harm. This is called a contra-indication. A family history of fits or convulsions may be a contra-indication against pertussis (whooping cough) vaccination, for example.

Limits on vaccines

Vaccines are made in ultra-sterile conditions in medical factories. They are distributed in their millions in ready-measured amounts or doses. Most are injected, preferably using sterile, one-use-only needles and syringes, by doctors or trained health workers. In some areas, people need to be told the benefits of immunization, by public health campaigns. But all this costs money, which is the main limit on immunization programmes in poorer countries.

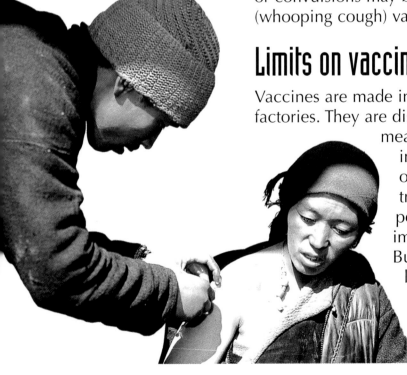

In some regions people are suspicious or distrustful of being injected with vaccines.

In the genes

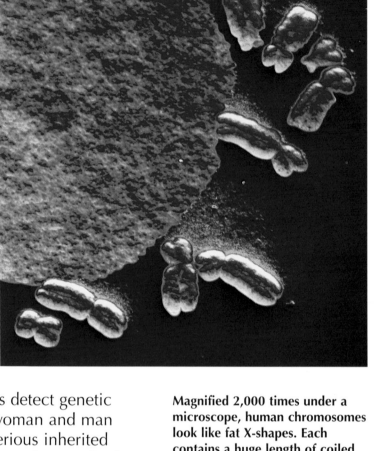

Each human body contains a set of around 100,000 instructions for making and running it. These are called 'genes' and they exist as codes of chemicals in the substance DNA (de-oxyribonucleic acid). Great lengths of DNA are twisted into 46 thread-like objects, chromosomes, found in nearly all the body's microscopic cells.

Genetic advice

A person's genes affect their resistance to disease, and also the likelihood of them developing some illnesses. Medical geneticists detect genetic problems and assess risks. For example, if a woman and man both come from families with a history of a serious inherited condition such as cystic fibrosis, they might consult a medical geneticist. This would help them to find out the chance of their unborn baby being affected.

Magnified 2,000 times under a microscope, human chromosomes look like fat X-shapes. Each contains a huge length of coiled DNA, bearing thousands of genes. The large 'ball' is the cell's nucleus, or control centre.

Medical geneticists use many techniques. A family history will be taken to record illnesses and conditions affecting parents and other relatives. This is because certain conditions are inherited in certain patterns. Chromosome analysis involves studying chromosomes directly, under a microscope. Some conditions are linked to a missing, extra or misshapen chromosome. In Down's syndrome, for instance, there are three chromosome 21s instead of the usual two.

Some genetic conditions

- **Haemophilia** Blood does not clot properly to seal a cut or wound.
- **Sickle-cell anaemia** Microscopic red blood cells become bent or sickled, blocking small blood vessels.
- **Cystic fibrosis** Sticky fluid builds up in the lungs.
- **Huntington's chorea** Loss of memory, and jerky movements.

Many other conditions, including certain types of heart disease, asthma, epilepsy and various cancers, have a genetic component. They tend to be inherited, but in a complex way that is only just being investigated.

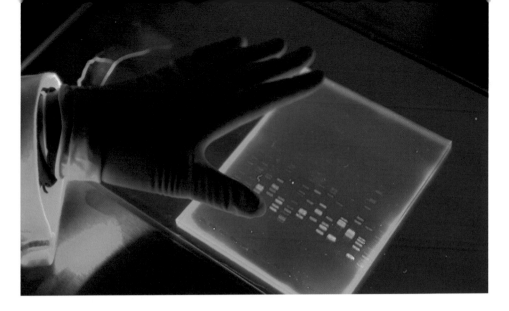

DNA fingerprints

The recent advance of 'genetic fingerprinting' uses cells containing DNA, taken as a sample. They are broken open and added to substances called enzymes. These snip the huge lengths of DNA into shorter pieces or fragments. More enzymes, called polymerases, make millions of copies of the DNA fragments in the PCR – polymerase chain reaction. This provides enough DNA for the technique of gel electrophoresis, which gives a pattern of dark bands – the genetic or DNA fingerprint or profile. It is unique to each individual, and possibly reveals genetic abnormalities which could cause illness.

Solutions and questions

DNA fingerprints are showing that more and more conditions – including being overweight, addicted or depressed – may be linked to genes. Identifying the genes may lead to treatment, even cure. But there are questions too. A baby's genes can be analysed before birth, from samples of blood or womb fluid. With so many types and chances of genetic problems, the decision to carry out a termination of pregnancy (abortion) gets ever more complicated.

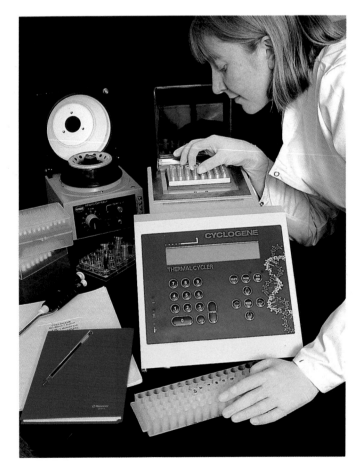

Right **Billions of multiple copies, or clones, of a tiny piece of DNA can be made by the polymerase chain reaction, in a machine that repeatedly warms and cools the chemicals.**

DIAGNOSING DISEASE

Diagnosis involves identifying a disease or condition from symptoms and signs so that it can be treated in the best way. Symptoms are problems the patient notices, such as a runny nose or a headache. Signs are features or changes that the doctor notices, such as an odd heartbeat sound or raised blood pressure.

Degrees of diagnosis

With a slight cold, it is not vital to pinpoint the exact germ responsible. Rest and hot, soothing drinks help natural recovery. But with serious conditions, speedy and accurate diagnosis allows correct treatment as soon as possible. Some of the greatest advances in diagnosis are due to high-tech engineering, making machines ever smaller, and controlling them with computers.

A protective screen shields the radiographer (imaging expert) from the patient having a chest X-ray. Standard or plain X-rays are still widely used, especially after injury, to diagnose broken bones and dislocated joints.

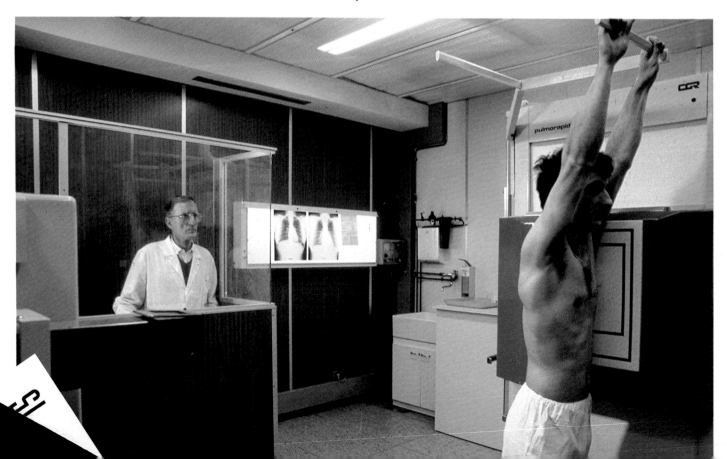

A bit of contrast

A standard X-ray shows very hard, dense body tissues, such as bone, cartilage and teeth, but not softer parts such as blood vessels and intestines. So a substance called a contrast medium is put into the body. This is radio-opaque, showing up white on X-ray to reveal the shape of the cavity or tube, and any blockage or abnormality. It is used in:

- **Angiogram** Arteries and veins, such as coronary angiography in the heart or cerebral angiography in the head
- **Arteriogram** Arteries only (see angiogram)
- **Barium enema** Last part of bowel
- **Barium meal** Stomach and intestine or bowel
- **Barium swallow** Gullet or oesophagus
- **Bronchogram** Bronchi and other branching airways in the lungs
- **Cholecystogram** Gall bladder and bile duct
- **Pyelogram** Kidneys, ureters (urine tubes) and bladder
- **Cystogram** Bladder

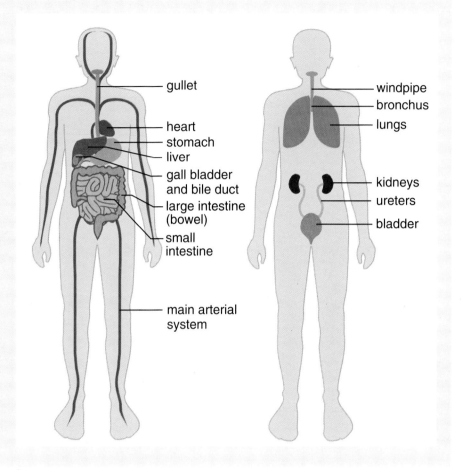

gullet
heart
stomach
liver
gall bladder and bile duct
large intestine (bowel)
small intestine
main arterial system

windpipe
bronchus
lungs
kidneys
ureters
bladder

Non-invasive diagnosis

Severe and repeated abdominal pain could have various possible causes. Previously, the main diagnostic method was to cut open the patient in an exploratory operation, to see inside. This type of invasive surgery carried its own risks, and there was no guarantee it would help.

Now there are many non-invasive methods, which do not involve cutting open the body. They include special X-ray machines, various scanners and imagers, electrical monitors that pick up the body's tiny electrical nerve signals, and tube-like endoscopes that go into natural body holes or tiny 'keyhole' incisions. Many of these methods are shown over the following pages. They would be impossible without computers to control the machinery, process the results, make wavy-line traces clearer, and sharpen and colour-enhance the pictures.

The age of the scanner

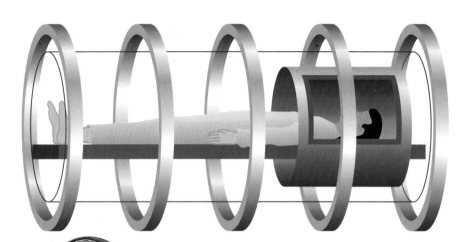

For an MR scan the patient lies in a giant washing-machine-like device that produces very strong magnetism. This makes the basic particles or atoms of body substances line up. Pulses of radio waves fired by the scanner through the body knock these atoms out of alignment. As they line up again, they give off their own tiny radio signals, which are detected by the machine's receivers.

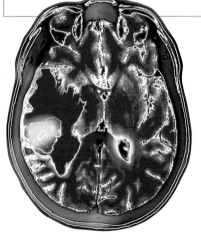

This computer-coloured MR scan of the head shows a view from above of a 'slice' through the brain, at eye level. The eyes are at the top of the image. The scan has revealed a brain growth or tumour, coded yellow, with a red damaged area around it.

The normal X-ray picture, or plain radiograph, is a 'snapshot' through the body. The coming of computers in the 1960s allowed medical scientists to make more detailed images, using X-rays and other waves. The speciality of radiology (taking X-rays) has widened into the huge area of medical imaging for diagnosis and treatment.

CT scans

The CT (computerized tomography) scan uses X-rays, but very weak and narrow-beamed, and so much less risky than a normal X-ray. The scanner beams them through the body many times at different angles. An array of sensors detects how much each beam is weakened by its passage through various tissues, such as bone and blood. A computer analyses the thousands of results and combines them to show a 'slice' of the body. It reveals much more detail than a normal X-ray, and many slices join into a three-dimensional image of the body's interior.

MRI scans

MRI (magnetic resonance imaging) also scans the body slice by slice. A computer processes the results to build up a detailed three-dimensional picture, even showing small nerves and blood vessels.

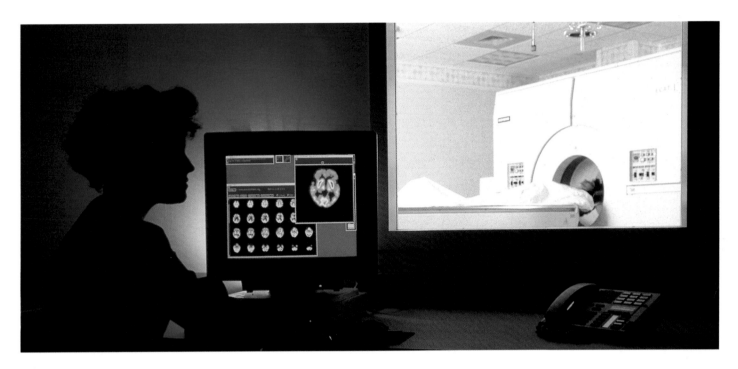

A PET scan

PET (positron emission tomography) shows not the structure of a part, but how 'busy' it is. Substances called radionuclides, that give off particles such as positrons, are put into the body. The scanner detects where they are concentrated and used.

Other types of radionuclide or radioisotope scans use different substances, which give off weak radioactivity. They move around the body and concentrate in certain parts, such as tumours (growths) or overactive glands (see also page 41).

The radiographer operates a PET scanner, as the patient lies on a table with her head inside the machine. The monitor screen shows computer-coloured images of the brain, indicating which parts are most active.

Seeing with sound

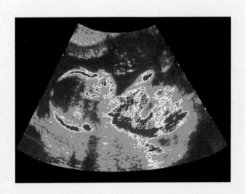

Ultrasound is high-frequency sound waves, far too shrill for us to hear. The microphone-shaped transducer emits ultrasound beams that enter the body, and its sensor picks up the different types of echoes from different parts and tissues. The all-important computer analyses the results into an image, the ultrasound scan, displayed on screen. Like MRI, ultrasound is harmless. It is used routinely to check developing babies in the womb. A specialized form, echocardiography, shows the heart beating 'live' on screen.

'Graphs and 'grams

The human body coordinates its movements and inner workings by its nervous system, with the brain in overall control. The system sends information in the form of electrical signals – nerve impulses. Millions of these whizz around the brain and body every second. Each lasts just a few thousandths of a second and has a strength of only one-twentieth of a volt.

Body tissues are actually about two-thirds water, and are therefore very good carriers, or conductors, of electricity. The 'echoes' of the electrical nerve impulses ripple through the tissues and flesh, and out to the skin. Here they can be picked up by sensors, and fed into electronic equipment which amplifies them. The signals are shown on a monitor screen or as wavy-line traces on paper. The pattern of the signals can help to identify problems or disease.

Specialized tests

There are many specialized diagnostic tests for eyes, ears, teeth and other body parts. For instance, after you have read letters on an eye chart, the ophthalmologist (eye specialist) may look into your eyes with a light-end-lens device, the ophthalmoscope. This shows the delicate blood vessels inside the eye, which can reveal general health or circulatory disorders. By bouncing air-jets off the eye from a puffer nozzle, the opthalmologist can show if the pressure inside the eyeball is unusually high or 'tense', which may signal glaucoma.

This young patient listens to different-pitched sounds, played through each headphone in turn. The test, pure-tone audiometry, helps to identify the extent and cause of hearing problems.

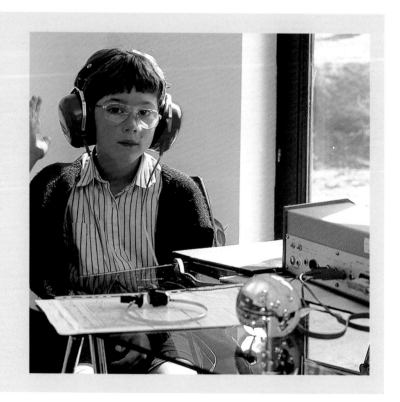

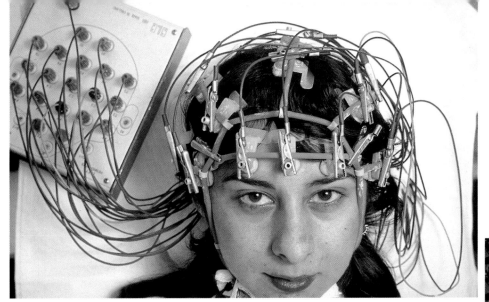

Brain-waves

The EEG (electro-encephalograph) machine detects nerve impulses from the brain that have passed out through the skull to the scalp skin. The resulting 'brainwaves' are called an electro-encephalogram. This can aid diagnosis, especially of various forms of epilepsy, encephalitis (brain inflammation) and meningitis, the effects of a stroke, brain tumours, and reasons for sleep disorders. The EEG trace is important when doctors are examining an unconscious person, because it can tell them how much brain activity there is and whether the person is 'brain dead', even though other body parts such as the heart may be active.

Heart traces

Sensors on the chest and arms can detect tiny electrical signals from the heart, which are fed into the ECG (electro-cardiograph) machine. These are displayed as an ECG trace, which may suggest various heart conditions, such as palpitations (irregular heartbeats), coronary disease, and even very minor heart attacks that hardly cause any symptoms.

An ECG can be done while a person rests on a couch, or walks, jogs or runs on a treadmill (see page 10). Alternatively, a small, portable ECG recorder (about the size of a mobile phone) strapped to the waist, can record the heartbeat continuously over a 24-hour period.

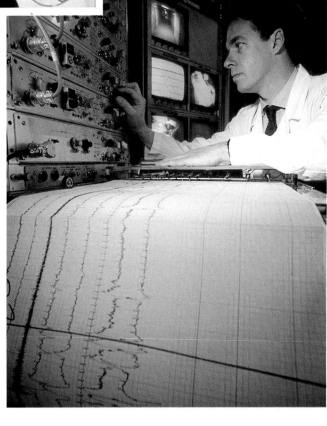

The sensors or electrodes of the EEG machine pick up the brain's own tiny electrical signals. The electrodes, on straps, are usually attached with paste or jelly, which easily wipes off (top picture). The procedure is totally painless. The signals are passed to a computer which enhances and displays them as a series of wavy-line traces, the electro-encephalogram (above).

Peering into the body

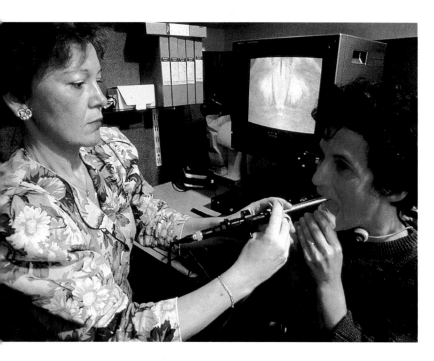

A doctor uses a laryngoscope to view the vocal cords, the white V-shaped strips on the screen, inside the patient's larynx or voice-box.

An endoscope enables a doctor to look directly into the body, rather than at a picture of the body on an X-ray or scan. This tube-like device is pushed inside the body, using natural body openings and passageways. Or it may be inserted through a tiny incision, for 'keyhole' diagnosis and treatment (see page 32). The patient may receive a local anaesthetic before endoscopy, to dull any discomfort.

Using an endoscope, the doctor can observe any problems, such as malformations, blood clots or other blockages, sore and raw spots and ulcers, growths and constrictions. Measurements can also be taken, for example, of blood pressure and oxygen content inside the heart. Sometimes, treatment is carried out at the same time, such as sealing an ulcer with laser light.

Names for 'scopes

Endoscopes have various designs, for different body parts.
- **Gastroscope** Down the throat and oesophagus (gullet), into the stomach, and perhaps farther into the intestine
- **Laryngoscope** Into the larynx (voice-box) in the neck
- **Bronchoscope** Down the windpipe into the bronchi and other lung airways
- **Colonoscope** Up the anus, up into the large intestine or colon
- **Sigmoidoscope and proctoscope** Up the anus, into the lower end of the digestive tract
- **Arthroscope** Into a joint, such as the knee or shoulder
- **Cystoscope** Up the urethra (urine tube) to the bladder, and perhaps farther, into the kidney
- **Sinuscope** Through the nose into the sinuses (air spaces in the skull) and internal ear
- **Laparoscope** Inside the abdomen

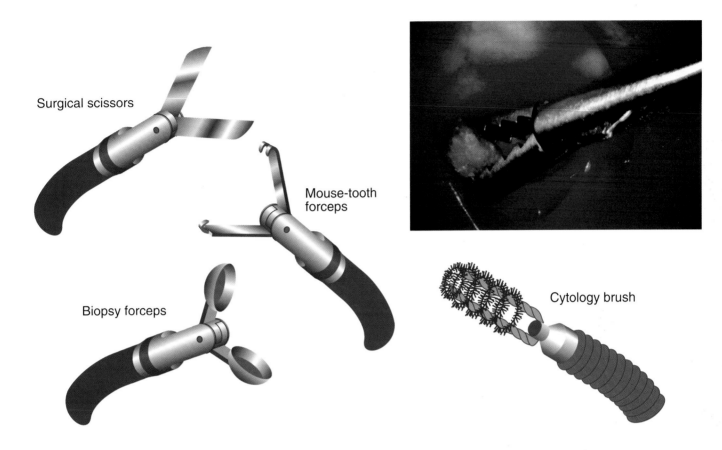

Surgical scissors

Mouse-tooth forceps

Biopsy forceps

Cytology brush

Multi-channels

Older endoscope designs were rigid, like thin telescopes. Newer versions are slim and flexible, and can be steered around the body's interior. An endoscope thinner than a drinking straw may have several tunnels or channels inside it:
• The lighting channel, carrying high-power or laser light to the tip. (It is dark inside the body!)
• The imaging channel, with a fibre-optic of more than 10,000 strands, or even a miniature TV camera.
• Steering channels, to flex the tip around corners or junctions.
• Working channels, to pump in air or fluid, since many body passages are usually squashed shut and need inflating for a clear view. These channels may also be used to pump in drug solutions, suck out samples of body fluid for analysis, or convey laser light for surgical incisions.
• A tiny pair of biopsy tweezers or grabs at the tip to grasp and remove a tissue sample for analysis, or a miniature baro-sensor to measure pressure.

The endoscope contains many different channels (described on the left). The range of instruments that can be attached to or passed down it includes:
• the biopsy forceps that nip out and hold on to a tiny piece of tissue (biopsy sample)
• cytology brush that rubs loose cells off a surface and retains them for analysis
• mouse-tooth forceps for grasping and removing objects
• surgical scissors for cutting off small growths.

The photograph shows a kidney stone being grasped by alligator forceps.

In the lab

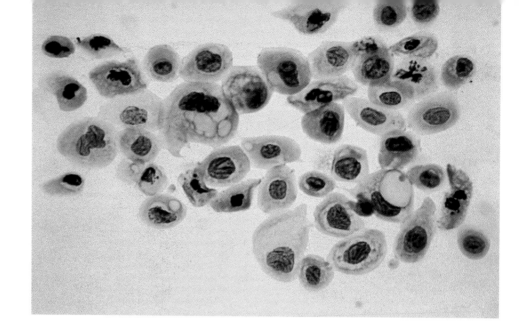

Under the microscope, cervical smear cells (from the cervix, or neck of the womb) stain a blue colour and contain large, dark nuclei (control centres). This indicates that they are becoming cancerous. Early treatment can remove the danger.

A large hospital has dozens of medical workers who are never seen by the patients but who are essential to the patients' well-being. They work in medical laboratories such as the 'path (pathology) lab' – with its shelves of chemicals, rows of test tubes, and busy, white-coated medical technicians. Much of the work is now carried out automatically by computer-controlled machines, which process thousands of samples every hour. One of the lab's main jobs is to analyse samples of fluids and tissues taken from patients (see page 11).

Methods of analysis

There are hundreds of lab tests for these different samples. Living cells may be cultured – grown in special nutrient mixtures – inside incubators. The cells are then stained (coloured) and examined under the microscope for signs of disease and other abnormalities. This technique is known as cellular pathology.

The unborn baby

A baby in the womb is not out of reach of diagnostic tests. In amniocentesis, a long hollow needle is inserted through the mother's body wall and womb, into the pool of fluid around the baby. This contains cells and chemicals from the baby's body, which can be withdrawn and tested for genetic and other disorders. In uterine villus sampling a needle is inserted along the birth canal, to take a sample of the baby's blood flowing through the placenta. Using such tests, doctors can plan treatment, or even carry out an induced or caesarean birth, to save the baby.

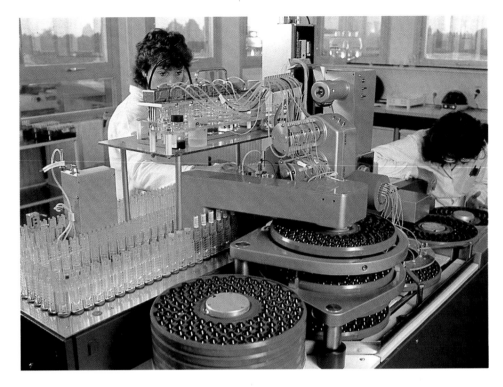

Automatic machinery has speeded up the analysis of samples taken from patients. It has also freed the medical technicians to concentrate on more tricky cases, and carry out more research and development.

If the doctors suspect that the patient has an infection, the sample taken from the patient may be treated in such a way as to encourage the germs in it to grow. The staff in the pathology laboratory can then precisely identify the germ and the doctor can decide how best to fight it. Antibiotic drugs may be tested against the germs in the laboratory to check that they are going to be effective before they are given to the patient.

Sterile conditions and other precautions are vital in the 'path lab'. This prevents the laboratory staff being infected by the samples they are testing – and the other way round, too.

Haematology

Blood is so important that it has its own branch of medicine, haematology. The number and shape of microscopic cells in a tiny sample of blood may suggest disease. Chemical tests measure the levels of hundreds of different substances in blood, such as oxygen, carbon dioxide, glucose (sugar), hormones, vitamins, antibodies and clotting factors. These procedures can reveal conditions such as anaemias, leukaemias, and haemophilia.

Testing, testing, testing . . .

- On average, each person in the USA has at least 20 medical laboratory tests each year.
- However these tests are concentrated mainly on patients in hospital. About half the population has no tests at all.
- The most common body substance analysed is blood, followed by urine.

EMERGENCY MEDICINE

Until the last 200 years emergency medicine was frequently worse than no medicine at all. Doctors had the best of intentions but they carried out procedures that were based on fashion, hearsay and unquestioned tradition, rather than scientific understanding.

Saved at the scene

In the twentieth century, one of medicine's great advances has been our understanding of what goes wrong with the body in medical emergencies, and how to take swift, life-saving action. This knowledge is helped by mobile phones and other up-to-date communications, modern rescue methods, new portable medical equipment and fast-acting drugs. Added to this is speedy transportation, first of paramedics to the patient, then of the patient to the medical centre. The chances of surviving a medical emergency are 20 times greater at the end of this century, than at the start.

The paramedic team set up a roadside operating theatre, at a major traffic accident. Trained surgeons use their mobile equipment, aided by other emergency workers. If they waited until the patient arrived at hospital, it would be too late.

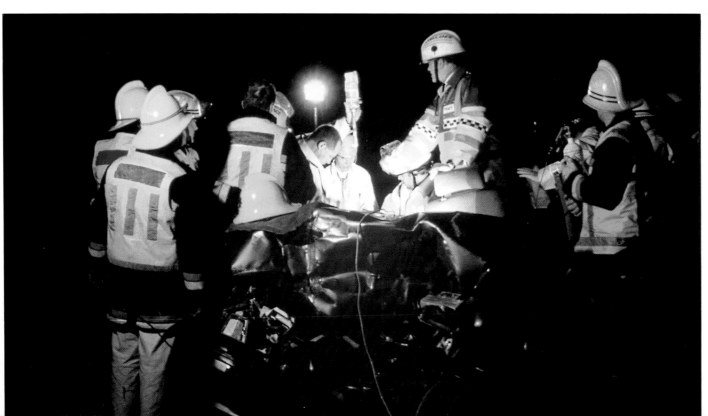

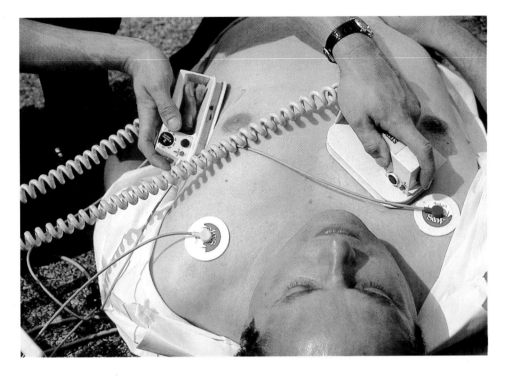

The cardiac defibrillator's two metal pads, electrodes, are placed on the chest and high-powered electricity passed between them. This aims to jolt the heart back into a steady beat. Defibrillation is used for a range of heart disorders, including heart attacks. The smaller circular electrodes are linked to an ECG machine.

Basic principles

The principles of first aid are to save life, to prevent the casualty's condition from getting worse, and to promote healing. Everyone is encouraged to learn something of first aid, since even the simplest action can help save a life. In most developed countries, expert medical help can be on the scene in minutes, so untrained helpers are advised to do the basic minimum in the meantime.

Watch and wait

In a typical heart attack, unless the person is in a very remote place, the recommended action is usually to call the emergency services, and keep the sufferer comfortable until help arrives. A modern ambulance is equipped with strong, rapid-action heart drugs such as adrenaline, replacement blood fluids, and a defibrillator, which uses electricity to 'shock' a trembling or fibrillating heart back into a steady beat. Medical advice can be given over the phone as necessary.

Less is more

If someone falls from a height, or is involved in a road traffic accident, or a sports injury, it is unwise to try and get them up and about, or to put on makeshift splints. Moving an already-damaged neck, back or limb could cause further damage, especially to the nerves, which may never heal. The usual action is to call for emergency help, and make the victim comfortable in the position he or she is in, until the experts arrive.

Intensive care

ew places have so much high-technology machinery as a hospital's intensive care unit (ICU). Patients here have life-threatening injuries, or serious medical emergencies such as heart attack or acute (sudden) kidney failure. The doctors, nurses and other staff are trained and qualified in the medical specialism of intensive care.

Monitoring the patient

Some equipment monitors the patient's condition, so doctors have early warning of further problems. Sensors and electrodes on the body continually detect body temperature, heart rate, blood pressure, breathing rate and other 'vital signs'. These are analysed by computer and displayed on a monitor screen. At a glance, staff can see the patient's overall condition. The computer beeps or flashes a warning if the signs alter.

The crash trolley

With so many ill people in hospital, a patient may suffer a medical emergency such as a heart attack anywhere, anytime. Crash trolleys are kept at certain authorized locations, ready for instant use. Each trolley has a selection of life-saving equipment, such as a cardiac defibrillator to re-start the heart by giving it an electric shock, various airways and drip lines, and large needles to inject powerful, fast-acting drugs exactly where the body needs them. The equipment is checked and replaced regularly, as necessary.

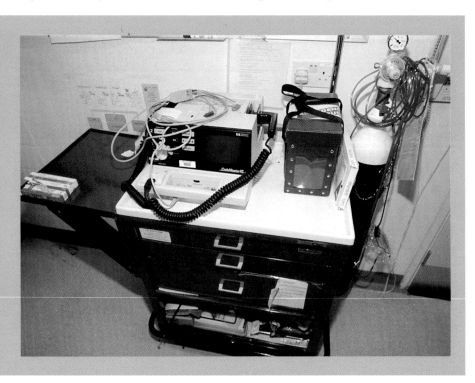

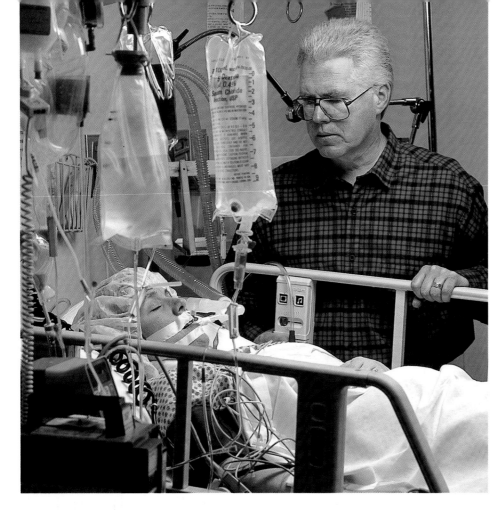

More than a dozen tubes and wires link the critically ill patient to an array of monitors and life-support equipment. Hanging up in the foreground are drip sachets and bags containing various fluids and drug solutions.

Supporting life

The ICU's life-support equipment includes 'drips', where liquids such as blood plasma or saline (a solution of balanced salts, like body fluid) are put into the body, usually via a needle inserted in an arm vein. These fluids replace fluids lost, for example, by severe bleeding or copious diarrhoea. Drugs can also be given through drip lines. Mouth or nasal tubes into the stomach may also convey fluids, nutrients and certain drugs.

If the patient has trouble breathing enough oxygen from normal air, an airway into the throat may carry almost pure oxygen gas. Oxygen can also be 'topped up' by a tube through the nose. For patients who cannot breathe properly on their own, an artificial ventilator can force a mixture of gases into and out of the lungs.

Special-care baby units

Some hospitals have intensive care facilities for very premature (early-born) or ill babies. These are NICUs, neo-natal intensive care units. The airways, injection needles and other items of equipment are much smaller, for the tiny patients. The latest 'smart-cot' incubator keeps the baby warm and in a controlled atmosphere, and monitors its vital signs. Movement sensors even monitor the baby's breathing motions, and warn staff if this falters.

SURGERY AND OPERATIONS

Right **An intense beam of red laser light shines from a laser scalpel. Different types of lasers are used to make beams for various jobs, such as removing birthmarks and other skin blemishes, or making extremely precise incisions (cuts) in body tissues.**

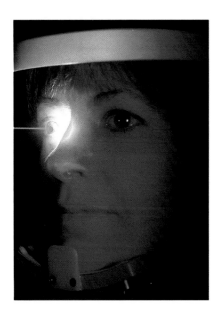

Above **A laser with green light shines into the eye, to carry out procedures such as sealing tiny leaking blood vessels.**

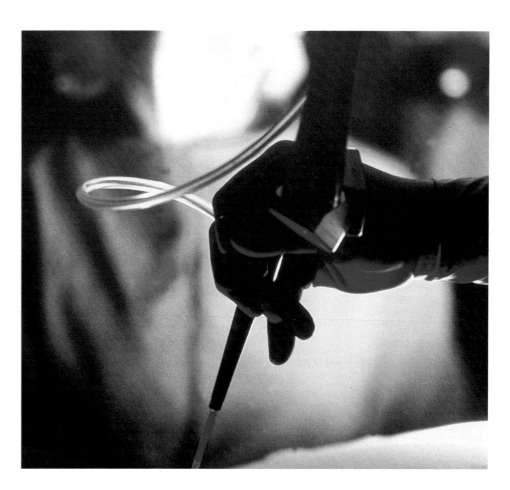

Surgery originally meant 'treating disease with the hands'. It has a very long and varied history. Many well-known names in medicine were surgeons who learnt their knowledge, skill and 'craft' on the battlefield. They were hailed as miracle-workers by some people, but as cruel butchers by others.

Cutting with light

Modern surgery uses the latest machines and technology to cause less and less trauma, or 'damage', to the body. The laser-scalpel's controlled beam of laser light can be accurately adjusted in width, depth and power, and focused to cut deeper tissues while leaving surface ones untouched. Its heat also 'welds' tiny blood vessels, to reduce bleeding. This makes laser-scalpels especially suitable for very delicate surgery, on the eyes, small nerves and similar fragile parts.

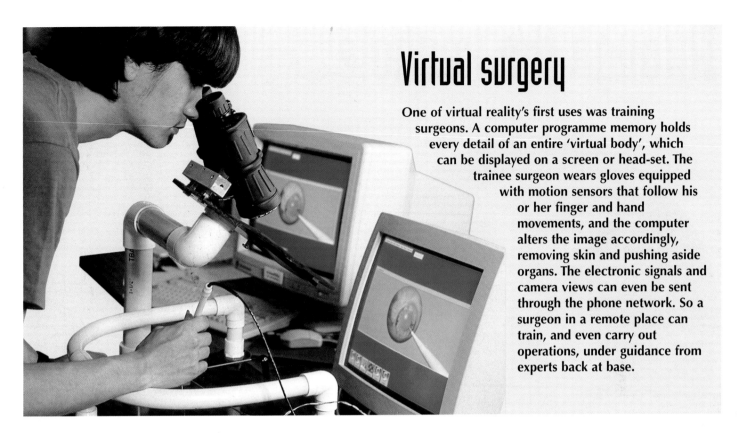

Virtual surgery

One of virtual reality's first uses was training surgeons. A computer programme memory holds every detail of an entire 'virtual body', which can be displayed on a screen or head-set. The trainee surgeon wears gloves equipped with motion sensors that follow his or her finger and hand movements, and the computer alters the image accordingly, removing skin and pushing aside organs. The electronic signals and camera views can even be sent through the phone network. So a surgeon in a remote place can train, and even carry out operations, under guidance from experts back at base.

Under the micro-knife

Microsurgery uses a high-powered binocular (two-eyed) microscope to see tiny nerves, blood vessels and other parts. The scalpels and other tools may be manipulated by a system of levers and gears in a frame, so that it is possible to move them by very small, precise amounts. This allows the surgeon to cut and join structures thinner than a hair with great precision, even reconnecting nerves so that the patient regains some movement and feeling in an accidentally amputated part.

Cold sleep

Anaesthesia, removing all feeling and sensation, has also progressed greatly. Modern local anaesthetic drugs are very accurate and effective, deadening only the part for surgery. This removes the need for a general anaesthetic, or putting the patient to sleep, which carries a small risk of complications. Better general anaesthesia and monitoring, along with cooling the body to about 6°C to slow its functions, means surgeons have more time for complex procedures. The cardiopulmonary, or heart-lung, machine takes over the jobs of breathing and pumping blood, so the surgeon can operate on the heart itself.

• In countries such as Britain, France and Australia, each person undergoes, on average, one surgical procedure per year.
• The longest operation was carried out in 1951 in Chicago, USA. It took 96 hours to remove a cyst (fluid-filled growth) from a woman's ovary.

Through the keyhole

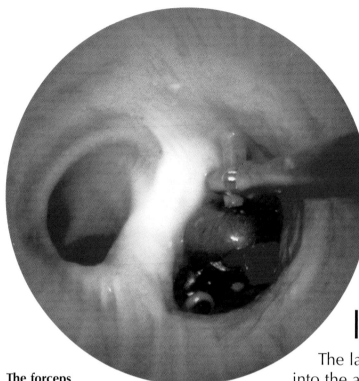

The forceps are trying to grab a plastic object, which a young child has accidentally breathed into its windpipe.

Surgery, like diagnosis, is becoming less invasive all the time. Endoscopes not only detect internal problems such as growths and ulcers. They can also carry out treatments, such as heat-sealing or cauterizing a blood leak, using high-power laser light or a hot electric-wire loop. Other endoscope attachments include tiny scalpels, forceps and other surgical instruments, to cut off growths or grab and remove foreign bodies (see page 23).

Inside the abdomen

The laparoscope is an endoscope designed to look into the abdomen, at the intestines, bladder, reproductive organs and other parts. It is inserted through a small 'keyhole' incision. After examining the scene, the surgeon may carry out surgical procedures such as cautery, using its working channels.

Micro-robots in the body?

Nano-technology deals with machines and devices that are microscopic, or even smaller! This may revolutionize medicine. Tiny nano-robots injected or swallowed into the body could be guided by remote control to the site of a growth, blood clot or other problem. The robot would treat the problem with drugs, miniature surgical instruments or radiation, and be recovered later.

Reproductive problems

The laparoscope is especially useful for fertility problems in women. Cysts and other growths may affect the ovaries (egg-containing glands). Inflammation and scar tissue may block the oviducts (fallopian tubes), along which ripe eggs travel on their way to the womb. Using a laparoscope, the gynaecologist can diagnose and perhaps treat such conditions.

The laparoscope is also used to gather ripe eggs, as they are released from the ovary and before they enter the oviduct, for in-vitro fertilization.

Adaptable catheters

A catheter is a long, thin, flexible tube. It is inserted into the body through a natural opening or small skin cut, and used to withdraw samples, inject liquids and drugs, take measurements or carry out treatments. It can be steered along blood vessels or between organs, as the doctor watches it 'live' on a monitor screen. It can also inject the contrast medium needed for certain types of X-rays (see page 17).

For heart problems, the catheter is inserted though a small incision in the groin, and threaded up a large vein to the heart. It may take blood samples or measurements, or introduce drugs. The balloon catheter's small, sausage-shaped tip is inflated to widen and unclog blocked blood vessels.

This patient is being treated by cardiac angioplasty. This involves threading a thin tube or catheter through a small skin incision, along blood vessels into the heart, while watching its progress on a monitor screen. The catheter shows up clearly as a curved dark line, although the heart itself is invisible. At the site of a blockage or narrowing in the blood vessel or heart valve, the catheter's tip is inflated with water like a small balloon, to widen the obstruction.

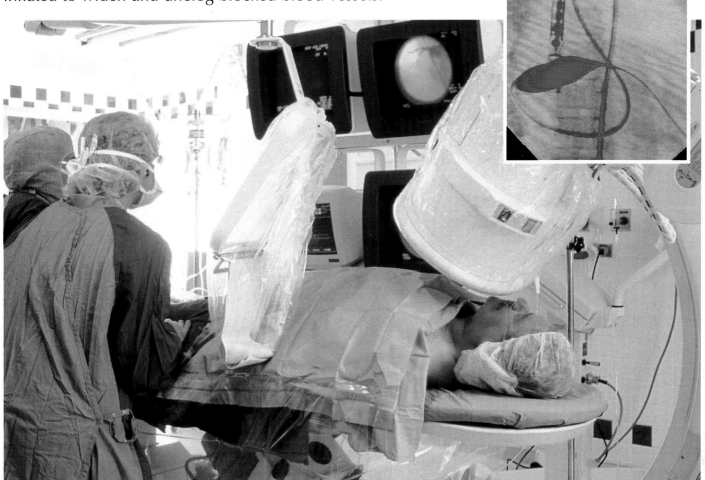

Transplants and implants

- A transplant is the transfer of a living part, such as a heart or kidney, from one person (or animal), called the donor, to another, the recipient.
- An implant is an artificial working part or other object inserted into the body.
- A prosthesis is an artificial, usually structural, part for the body.

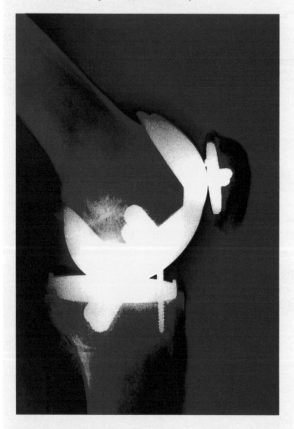

This computer-coloured X-ray shows an artificial knee joint, in yellow, including the screw that fixes the lower part onto the top of the shin bone. Artificial joints usually replace joints damaged by various forms of arthritis or rheumatism, or by over-use or injury.

Transplants

Transplants were first tried in the 1600s when doctors transferred blood from a person or animal, into a patient. Unfortunately, the patient invariably died. In the 1900s Austrian scientist Karl Landsteiner discovered different blood groups: A, B, AB and O. Now blood, tissues and organs are used that match the recipient's group as closely as possible. This reduces the chances of the patient's body rejecting the transplanted part.

Suppressing rejection

Since the 1980s, the problems of rejection have been lessened by a new generation of drugs, the immuno-suppressives. They damp down the body's immune system, which normally fights invading germs and also causes rejection. Their use means a transplant is more likely to 'take'. Like most drugs, however, they have side-effects. Because they lessen resistance to germs, they make infections more likely.

What is transplanted?

The modern era of transplants began in the 1950s with kidneys. Today's transplants include the heart, lungs and liver (sometimes in combination), heart valves, kidney, pancreas, bone marrow, skin, and the cornea and lens in the eye. There are many people waiting to be recipients of a transplant, but there is a shortage of donors in suitable medical condition (usually road-traffic accident victims), with suitable permission from relatives.

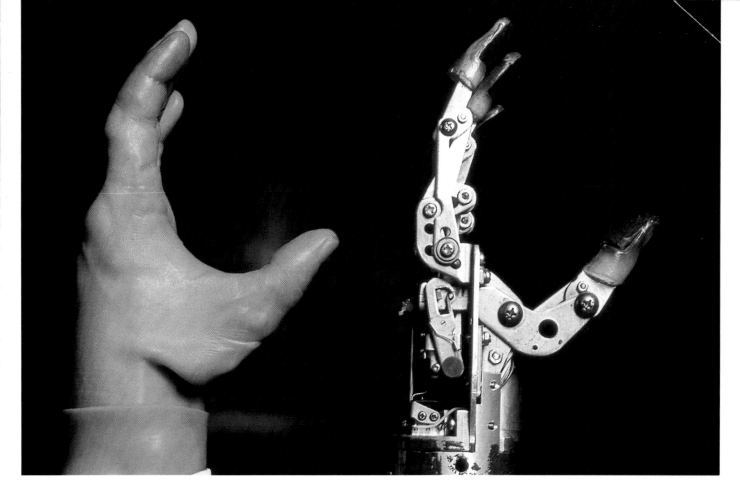

Implants and prostheses

Among the oldest known artificial body parts are false teeth of wood, gold and ivory, from Ancient Rome. With modern materials, medical technologists are producing greatly improved implants. They include eye lenses, tiny stirrup bones in the ear, plastic blood vessels and lung airways, valves in the heart, heart-assist pumps, metal pins, strips and plates for broken bones, and metal-and-plastic artificial joints, such as the hip, shoulder, elbow and knuckle.

Working artificial hands have sensors to detect nerve signals in the user's skin. These control tiny motors that move the fingers, which bear touch-sensors so they do not crush fragile items. This realistic-looking hand was produced using techniques from robotics and electronics.

Bio-inert materials

Any object that gets into the body may trigger the immune defence system, which tries to destroy and reject it. This happens equally with a germ, a splinter jabbed through the skin, or an implanted artifical part, such as a heart valve or joint. Bio-engineers are continually searching for materials and substances which are more 'biologically inert', or inactive. They are designed to avoid triggering the body's defences. They include various types of plastics, like teflon, and stainless steel and other metals.

DRUGS AND RADIATION

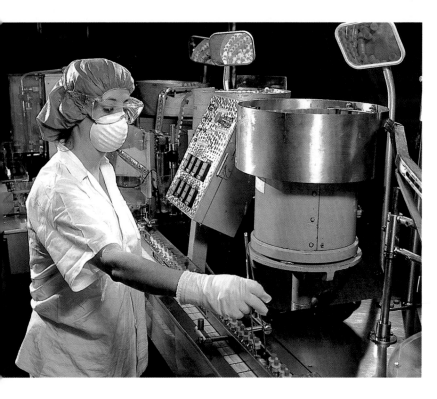

Drugs are made and packaged in ultra-clean factory-laboratories. Workers carefully watch and double-check the automatic equipment. Every container has a batch code so that it can be traced, in case of problems.

Surgery is only one type of medical treatment. Other types include physical therapies, such as heat treatment, manipulation and exercises (physiotherapy), chemical therapies, which use drugs made from natural sources or in the laboratory, and radiation therapies, such as X-rays, known as radiotherapy.

Traditional drug sources

In ancient times people discovered that chewing a certain plant might relieve a headache or abdominal pain. From these observations grew the skills of herbalists and apothecaries. There are still thousands of traditional remedies around the world prepared from natural substances – herbs and other plants, but also minerals in rocks and soils, and even animal products such as blood, urine, bile and bone. About half of modern, scientifically tested drugs are also still based on natural substances, especially on those extracted from plants.

Drugs from bugs

Genetic engineering and biotechnology are advancing drug production. For example, the gene for making a specific drug substance can be isolated from a plant, animal or microbe, and inserted into microbes such as *Escherschia coli* bacteria. These are grown in huge vats. The new genes instruct the microbes to make the required drug, which is then separated and purified. During the 1980s, the hormone called human insulin (used to treat diabetes) was made in this way, by microbes. Formerly, diabetic people used slightly different forms of insulin, from cows or pigs.

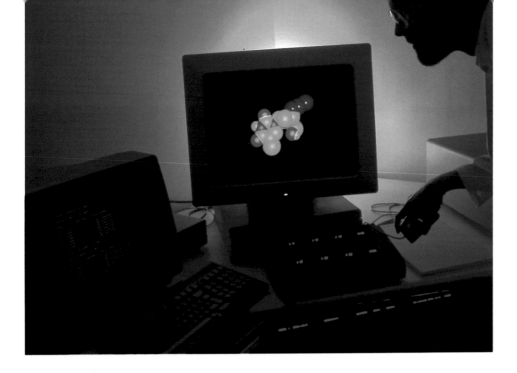

A computer program shows a three-dimensional 'space-filler' model of the structure of the drug AZT, used to treat AIDS. The different-coloured balls on the screen represent atoms such as carbon and hydrogen, within the drug molecule.

Computer chemotherapy

A growing number of drugs are not based on plant and animal substances. They are created, tested and altered in the laboratory. These artificial drugs are called chemotherapeutic agents, and some are known as 'designer drugs'. The structure of the drug's individual molecules is analysed by complex chemical tests, such as X-ray crystallography, spectrometry and chromatography. It can then be displayed as a three-dimensional model on a computer screen. The chemists, biologists and pharmacologists (drug scientists) work together to alter it in the smallest detail to improve its effects. The drugs called calcium blockers and beta blockers, for heart disease, have been improved in this way.

1 in 20,000

Laws in most countries say that any chemical intended to be a drug must be tested in turn on
- living cells in dishes
- certain animals
- volunteer humans in small-scale clinical trials.

Modern methods of tissue culture, growing cells in tubes and on plates, are reducing the need for some of the animal tests. At every stage, all side-effects and other problems are noted. Only 1 'hopeful' drug in 20,000 makes it through to general use.

Routes for drugs

The effect of a drug depends partly on its chemical structure. It also depends on the 'route of administration', which is the way it gets into the body, and where it goes once inside. There are dozens of new technologies for improving drug administration, making it more effective, safer and more convenient, and reducing side-effects.

Oral drugs

Pop a tablet into your mouth, and you are taking it by the oral route. Some drugs are made as capsules containing tiny particles, encased in various coatings. The different coatings are digested away at different rates in the stomach and intestines. These time-release capsules mean the drug is taken into the body at a steady rate, rather than in one large wave.

Topical drugs

A topical drug is applied directly to the affected area, for fast and local action. Skin creams and ointments are common examples. In a skin patch, the drug is contained on an adhesive patch, like a sticking plaster. It passes slowly through the skin, into the body. Drugs against angina (heart pain) and motion sickness, hormone replacement for women, and drugs to help people stop smoking, can be given by skin patch.

The pocket aerosol inhaler produces a fine spray of drug, breathed down into the lungs. It works 'topically' in the bronchi and bronchioles (airways), preventing them from narrowing or constricting. If the same drug was not given topically, but by tablet or injection, it would spread all over the body and have unwanted side-effects in other parts.

Drugs for breathing problems such as asthma can be given by pocket inhalers, or breathed in through a face mask from larger aerosol or nebulizer equipment. The tiny drug droplets go into the lungs, for fast and localized action.

38

Injections

'Hypodermic' means 'below the skin'. Hypodermic needles and syringes introduce a drug through the skin, directly into body tissues. In a depot injection, the drug is mixed with an inert or inactive substance that dissolves very slowly. It releases the drug gradually, over weeks or months. Or the drug can be implanted under the skin as a capsule. These methods reduce the need for lots of separate injections. They also help people who forget their regular injections – or avoid them.

Pumps and minipumps

The drug pump is a small, battery-powered device strapped to the body. It injects tiny, regular amounts of a drug, such as insulin, through a needle. The minipump is implanted under the skin. As watery fluid from body tissues passes naturally in through the casing into the pump, it pushes the drug slowly and steadily out into the tissues.

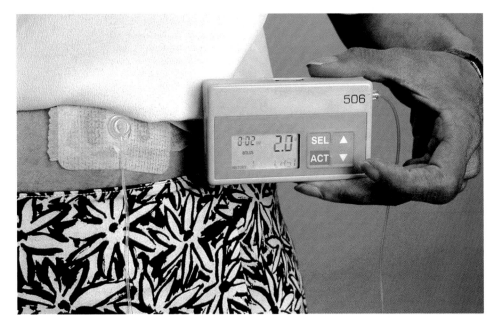

This portable insulin pump for diabetic people can be programmed to release the amount of insulin required by the wearer's body for different activities, such as eating a meal or taking exercise. The drug passes along the thin tube into the body through a needle under the dressing.

Rays that heal

The high-energy physics machine called a linear accelerator produces rays for radiotherapy, used to treat a small brain tumour. The rays are beamed in from different angles, so only the diseased part receives the accumulated, harmful dose. The metal frame holds the patient's head steady, for exact positioning.

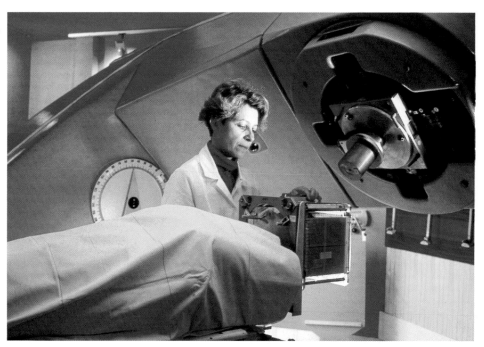

About the time X-rays were discovered, scientists also found that substances such as radium and uranium gave off invisible 'rays'. These various forms of rays and particles, known as radiation, were hailed as medical miracles. But within a few years, they were known to be the opposite. They have serious effects on microscopic body cells and living tissues, causing burns, radiation sickness, cancers and other health problems.

Radiotherapy

Gradually, physicists learned more about different kinds of radiation, and how to control them. Medical scientists discovered that suitably small amounts of radiation, applied to a small area such as a cancerous growth, could kill the microscopic cancer cells without affecting the surrounding parts. This is the basis of radiation therapy, or radiotherapy.

Which rays?

Most radiotherapy is for cancers. Because the rays can be so dangerous, treatment is tailored to each patient. Often, surgery and/or drug therapy are also given.

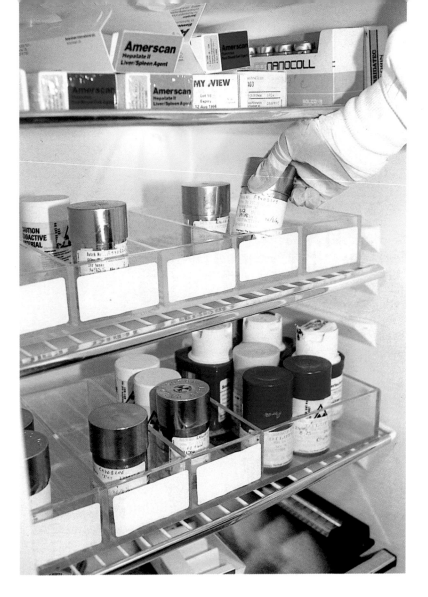

Radiation therapy uses beams of electrons (cathode rays), X-rays or gamma rays. These are produced by large machines such as linear accelerators (see panel). The patient lies on a treatment table and the rays are directed and focused so the radiation is concentrated in the diseased part. Lead sheets shield the rest of the body. The treatment may last a few minutes, every day or so for several weeks, but exact timings vary.

Isotopes and implants

Some body chemicals concentrate naturally in certain tissues or organs. For example, the substance iodine collects naturally in the thyroid gland, where it is used to make body hormones. A laboratory-made radioactive form, or radioisotope, of iodine collects here too. Its concentrated radiation can be used to kill a growth or tumour in the thyroid gland. Different radioisotopes are used to treat diseases in other organs.

The radiotherapy medicine cabinet contains various radioactive chemicals, as liquids and pellets, for injecting or implanting. Each is kept in its own radiation-proof container.

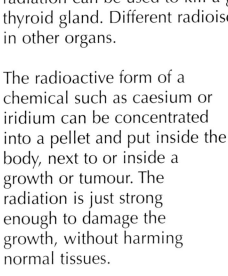

The radioactive form of a chemical such as caesium or iridium can be concentrated into a pellet and put inside the body, next to or inside a growth or tumour. The radiation is just strong enough to damage the growth, without harming normal tissues.

Physics and medicine

The accelerators, cyclotrons and other 'atom-smasher' machines which make high-energy radiation are extremely complex and costly. They are used by two groups of scientists. One is doctors called radiotherapists, and their patients. The other is particle physicists, who carry out research into the electrons and other particles which make up all matter in the Universe. Both groups share knowledge and benefits.

MEDICINE OF THE FUTURE

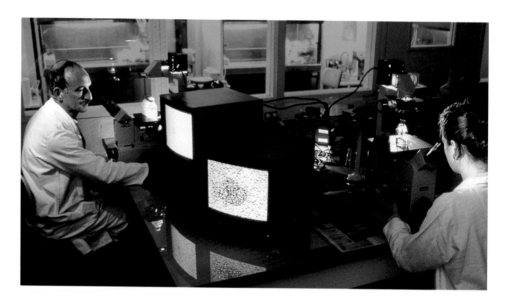

Scientists view microscopic white blood cells on monitor screens. It is part of the worldwide Human Genome Project, to identify all 100,000 human genes, where they are on the chromosomes inside cells – and how they cause inherited diseases.

The fight against disease

- In 1980 the disease smallpox was wiped out, after a worldwide campaign of health education and immunization.
- A similar campaign against malaria has been less successful. This disease still kills more than 2 million people yearly in tropical and subtropical places.
- As some diseases disappear, new ones appear. In 1981 the infection AIDS (Acquired Immune Deficiency Syndrome), caused by HIV (Human Immunodeficiency Virus), was recognized for the first time.

Every year brings greater advances in medicine. In particular, genetics offers many hopes for the future. Gene therapy aims to replace faulty genes with normal ones in people who have inherited diseases such as muscular dystrophy, haemophilia and sickle-cell anaemia. This would treat the cause, rather than the symptoms. However there are problems incorporating the normal genes into suitable body cells, which are always multiplying and dying.

New drugs also offer great hope against many diseases, but sometimes their bad effects are not obvious until years later. Drug research is immensely lengthy and costly, and some people disagree with the use of animals as 'guinea pigs'.

Better hi-tech engineering methods and electronics have many benefits for medicine. Scanning methods continue to improve. and specialist forms of surgery, such as minimally invasive techniques and microsurgery, are also progressing. Ever more miniature batteries, motors, circuits and similar devices are leading to better artificial implants and body parts.

Medical advances depend, however, not only on such technological developments, but on people's attitudes and values, and also on laws and guidelines, which can stop or slow down some areas of medical research.

Electronic bodies

The electronics and computing revolution also benefits patients. The similarity between the body's tiny electrical signals in its nerves and brain, and a computer's tiny electrical signals in its wires and microchips, mean that the two sciences have much in common. Computers with 'neural net' circuits are modelled on the workings of the nervous system, while electronic implants should help people with problems affecting the eyes, ears, nerves or brain.

Better health for fewer people

The overall result of these medical advances is that people live longer, healthier lives. But only some people. The latest medicine uses huge amounts of money, but it is spent on relatively few patients in the world. Some people feel that medical money should be spread more evenly and on more basic tasks, such as cleaner water, better food, immunization and publicity campaigns. These are effective ways of preventing disease among millions.

Advanced electronics are bringing implants into a new era. The cochlear implant's microchip circuits turn sounds into electrical signals, fed directly into the ear's nerves, to relieve deafness. The retinal implant (see page 5) may do the same inside the eye – allowing the blind to see.

It's up to us

Modern medicine seems to be miraculous. But even the latest high-technology medical care can only do so much. It is up to each person to eat suitable foods, take exercise, not smoke, generally follow a healthy lifestyle – and to report health problems to the doctor at an early stage. Better health and earlier diagnosis usually means less need for medicine!

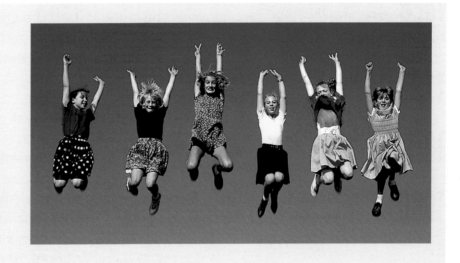

DATE CHART

400 BC In Ancient Greece Hippocrates describes basic methods and procedures in medicine, and founds the profession of physician.

180 AD In Ancient Rome Claudius Galen produces his summary of knowledge in anatomy and medicine.

1414 The infection of influenza is described for the first time, in Paris.

1543 In Padua, Italy, Andreas Vesalius rejects traditional teaching and founds the science of anatomy with his books *On the Structure of the Human Body*.

1596 In China the book *Ben-zao Gang-mu* describes more than 8,000 uses for medicines made from plants and animals.

1628 In England William Harvey demonstrates the circulation of the blood, pumped by the heart.

1796 In England Edward Jenner develops vaccination against smallpox.

1816 The stethoscope is invented.

1860s The sphygmomanometer, to measure blood pressure, and the clinical thermometer are developed.

1882 Robert Koch is first to show a definite link between a specific disease, tuberculosis, and a certain microbe or germ, the TB bacillus.

1896 The first X-rays for medical diagnosis are taken at Columbia University, USA.

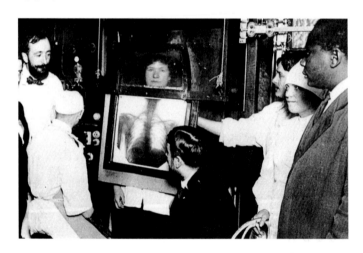

1903 German surgeon George Pethers suggests the use of X-rays to treat cancer (radiotherapy). William Einthoven invents the ECG machine.

1911 In London, William Hill invents the first gastroscope.

1929 German psychiatrist Hans Berger develops the first EEG machines. Fleming reports his discoverery of penicillin.

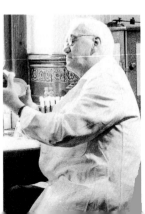

1938 The first artificial hip joints are implanted.

1940 Penicillin is first used to treat patients – soldiers wounded in World War II.

1943 Renal dialysis machines, or 'artificial kidneys' first used.

1952 George Jorgenson becomes Christine Jorgenson, in the first sex-change operation.

1953 American surgeon John Gibbon uses his cardio-pulmonary bypass machine, or 'heart-lung machine', for the first time.

1956 The first trials of the birth control pill for women, the 'Pill' oral contraceptive, begin in Puerto Rico.

1958 The first ultrasound scans are made, to check babies in the womb.

1962 The first laser surgery is carried out, on the eye.

1967 Christiaan Barnard carries out the first heart transplant.

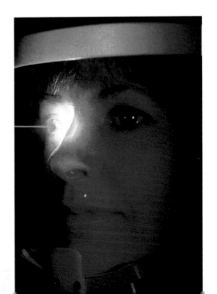

1973 The first CAT and MRI scanners are used on patients.

1978 The first 'test tube baby', conceived by in-vitro fertilization (IVF), is born in Britain.

1981 AIDS is officially recognized as a medical condition, by the US Centers for Disease Control, Atlanta.

1982 The first product of genetic engineering, human insulin (for treating diabetes) made by altered bacteria, goes onto the market.

1986 The first gene for an inherited disease, Duchenne muscular dystrophy, is identified.

1991 1 December is World AIDS Day, the first global medical event, to bring attention to the disease and its problems.

1994 Experiments with genetically engineered pigs aim to produce organs for transplant into humans.

1996 Tests begin on a contraceptive that prevents sperm formation in men.

1997 A female sheep is cloned from another adult as a genetic copy, making the use of animal organs for transplants, and animals as living drug factories more likely.

GLOSSARY

abdomen The stomach, intestines and surrounding area.

amplify To make stronger or more powerful, especially with electrical signals (as in a hi-fi music amplifier).

anaemias A group of conditions where the blood cannot carry enough oxygen around the body, usually due to problems with the oxygen-carrying substance haemoglobin in its microscopic red blood cells.

anaesthetic A substance or process that removes all sensations and feelings, especially touch and pain.

anatomy The study of the body's structure, including its organs and tissues. The study of the body's workings or functions is called physiology.

acupuncture Ancient Eastern technique of piercing the body with special needles at specific sites, to restore and re-balance its flow of life energy or *chi* essential for good health.

biopsy Removing a small portion of living tissue, such as a piece of a muscle, and testing it to help diagnosis.

complementary medicine A type or form of medicine which is not fully part of the modern scientific Western medicine, but which can be used alongside it and add to its effectiveness.

contrast medium A substance that shows up on X-ray, in order to outline body parts and tissues which do not normally show up.

gynaecologist Doctor who specializes in problems of the female reproductive organs and closely linked parts of the body.

haemophilia A 'bleeding disease' in which a person's blood does not clot properly to seal a cut or wound.

immune system Parts of the body which protect it by fighting invading germs and other 'foreign bodies'.

immunization Making the body resistant to attack by germs such as bacteria and viruses.

incision A cut or slice into the body, usually made on purpose, as in surgery.

infectious disease A disease where germs (harmful microbes) infect the body – that is, get inside and multiply and cause symptoms. Also, a disease that can be spread by germs.

invasive 'Invading' or getting into the body, usually through purpose-made incisions, as during an operation.

in-vitro fertilization (IVF) Involves taking ripe eggs from a woman and fertilizing them with sperm from a man. The resulting embryo is put back into the woman's womb where, hopefully, it develops normally.

leukaemias A group of cancer-like conditions of the blood, usually where the blood's microscopic white blood cells multiply out of control.

paramedics People who have medical training, especially in emergency medicine, who supplement the work of the medical profession, but who are not fully qualified doctors.

pathology The study of abnormal changes and diseases in the body, including what causes them,

and what happens during their development.
sterile Absence of living microbes, including germs.

volt Electricity's strength or pushing force. A torch or personal-stereo battery is usually 1.5 (one and a half) volts. Mains electricity from a wall socket is 240 volts.

FIND OUT MORE

Books to read

Eyewitness Science – Medicine by Steve Parker (Dorling Kindersley, 1995)
New Technology – Medicine and Health by Nigel Hawkes (Gloucester Press 1994)
A History of Medicine – From Prehistory to the Year 2020 by Nancy Duin and Dr Jenny Sutcliffe (Simon & Schuster 1992)
The Wayland Library of Science and Technology – The Human Machine by Brenda Walpole (Wayland, 1990)
The Human Body – series published by Wayland 1996–7

Places to visit

'Science for Life' at The Wellcome Institute, 183 Euston Road, London, UK (moving to Manchester in 1998)
World-famous collections of medical equipment and specimens, and regular special events.

Science Museum, Exhibition Road, London, UK
Occasional displays of medical equipment and methods.

Royal Museum of Scotland, Chambers Street, Edinburgh, UK
Some scientific and medical displays.

Thackray Medical Museum, Beckett Street, Leeds LS9 7LN
Realistic scenes showing how disease-ridden people were in historical times.

INDEX